Fasting: The Path to Health and Vitality

Discovering Ancient Wisdom for Modern Wellness

By

STEVE ROBINS

Table of contents

Introduction

Embracing the Excursion of Fasting

In a world set apart by persevering timetables and a steady deluge of food choices, the idea of fasting arises as a groundbreaking and old practice that holds the possibility to reform our way of dealing with well-being and imperativeness. "Fasting: The Path to Health and Vitality" digs into the profundities of this deeply rooted custom, revealing its significant effect on actual prosperity, mental lucidity, and profound enhancement. Go along with me on an excursion through the set of experiences, science, and speciality of fasting as I investigate how swearing off food can open a pathway to restoration, versatility, and re-established captivation.

In this basic part, I leave on a journey to grasp the quintessence of fasting and its pertinence in our cutting-edge lives. We will strip back the layers of time to uncover how societies across the ages have embraced fasting for food as a useful asset for mending and self-revelation. As I set up our investigation, I welcome you to open your brain and heart to the conceivable outcomes that lie ahead. Whether you are an inquisitive rookie or a carefully prepared professional, this book means to give you experiences, direction, and motivation as you set out on your very own excursion along the way to well-being and essentialness through fasting.

Chapter One

The Authentic Embroidery: Fasting Across Societies and Times

Fasting, with its underlying foundations profoundly woven into the texture of mankind's set of experiences, has been rehearsed across assorted societies and ages. In this part, we navigate the

records of time to uncover the richly embroidered artwork of fasting rehearsals that have spread over landmasses and ages. From old civilizations to present-day times, fasting has
had a significant impact on strict customs, philosophical pursuits, andwell-being customs.
We dive into the acts of fasting among the ancient Egyptians,Greeks, and Romans, where fasting was interwoven with otherworldliness and venerated to purge both body and soul. Investigating the strict meaning of
fasting in Judaism, Christianity, Islam, Hinduism, and Buddhism, we reveal the shifting translations and practices that have been passed down through hundreds of years.
This section additionally reveals insight into outstanding
authentic figures who embraced fasting, from profound pioneers to logicians,who outfitted its groundbreaking potential to accomplish illumination,self-control, and unwavering focus. As we venture through time, we experience occasions where fasting was utilised as a type of dissent, backing, and social change.
Through these verifiable tales and diverse correlations, we gain a more profound appreciation for fasting's role as a channel for self-revelation, inward strength, and association with the heavenly. Go along with us as we disentangle the strings of fasting's authentic embroidery,
winding around together the tales, customs, and insights that keep on moulding how we might interpret this old practice.
Fasting is a string that winds through the texture of mankind's set of experiences, interfacing with civic establishments and ages across the globe. In this section, we dig into the rich woven artwork of fasting,uncovering their assorted social settings and the significant effect they've had on social orders over time.

Section 2.1: Old Insight and Ceremonies
- The underlying foundations of fasting in old human advancements: Mesopotamia, Egypt, and then some.

- Fasting as an Otherworldly Practice: Experiences from Buddhism,Hinduism, and Jainism.
- Abrahamic customs: Fasting in Judaism, Christianity, and Islam.

Section 2.2: Fasting For Mending and Change

-Greek and Roman viewpoints: Fasting for physical and mental prosperity.

-Monks and spiritualists: Fasting as a way to edification and self-acknowledgement.

-Native customs: Fasting in local societies and its association with nature

Section 2.3: Fasting In the Cutting-Edge Age

-Fasting amid a shortage: Authentic and wartime viewpoints.

- Renaissance and Edification Impacts: Changing Views of Fasting.

-Contemporary resurgence: The recovery of fasting in advanced health development.

As we unwind the tales of fasting's part in various social orders, you'll come to see the value in how this antiquated practice has advanced, adjusted, and formed human encounters over hundreds of years. Go along with us on this enrapturing venture through time and gain a more profound comprehension of the social importance and significance of fasting as a way to well-being and imperativeness.

Throughout the records of time, fasting has woven itself into the texture of different societies and ages, serving not just as an act of confidence and self-restraint but additionally as a channel for physical and profound change. In this part, we dig into the different types of fasting customs that have arisen across the globe, spreading from antiquated civilizations to the present day.

We'll travel back to ancient Egypt, where fasting was interlaced with ceremonies of purging and association with the heavenly. We'll investigate the fasting practices of Buddhist priests, whose abstention from strong food was viewed as a way to develop care and separation. Wandering into bygone eras, we'll reveal how fasting was seen during strict observances in Christianity and Islam, conveying emblematic implications of penance and commitment. As we navigate through history, we'll experience fasting presence in native societies, where it was a method for regarding predecessors and outfitting otherworldly energy. From Local American vision missions to Hindu fasting during celebrations, every custom divulges a one-of-a-kind feature of fasting's significant effect on the human experience.

This section fills in as an entryway to the past, enlightening how fasting's importance has developed and adjusted across social scenes. By understanding the underlying foundations of these practices, we gain a more profound appreciation for the unpredictable connection between fasting, human convictions, and the quest for prosperity. Go along with us as we disentangle
the strings that fasten the richly embroidered artwork of mankind's set of experiences.

Chapter Two

Exploring Healthful Science: What Fasting Means for the Body

In the mind-boggling dance between food and well-being, fasting arises as an enthralling accomplice that coordinates an orchestra of physiological changes inside the human body. This part digs into the domain of
healthy science, looking beneath the surface to uncover the mind-boggling systems through which fasting applies its

extraordinary impact. We set out on an excursion through the body's reactions to fasting, investigating the intriguing interaction between chemicals, digestion, and cell restoration.

Diving into the universe of autophagy, we uncover how fasting prompts the body's self-cleaning systems, getting out damaged cells and making them ready for restoration.

From the long periods of tracker finders to the state-of-the-art bits of knowledge of present-day research, we follow the advancement of how we might interpret fasting's effect on weight, insulin responsiveness, and general life span. We'll investigate the science behind discontinuous fasting and broadened diets and their likely advantages for cerebrum wellbeing,cardiovascular capability, and even disease anticipation.

Amid the ocean of logical disclosures, we'll likewise explore the shores of wariness, revealing insight into possible dangers and contemplations while leaving on a fasting venture. With a compass directed by proof and exploration, this section outfits you with a more profound cognizance of how fasting, as a revered practice, interweaves with the mind-boggling ensemble of the human body's complicated symphony. Go along with us as we explore the flows of nourishing science and disclose the musical agreement of fasting's effect on well-being and essentialness.

Inside the unpredictable hardware of the human body, fasting triggers a fountain of physiological reactions that reach a long way beyond simple cravings for food. In this section, we dive into the domain of wholesome science to reveal the mind-boggling manners in which fasting influences our science and prosperity.

We'll leave on an excursion through the metabolic scene,investigating how fasting starts cycles, for example, autophagy, where cells

participate in self-purging systems, and ketosis, where the body moves to consume fat for fuel. We'll dig into the many-sided dance of chemicals, uncovering what fasting means for insulin awareness, chemical emission

development, and the sensitive equilibrium of energy homeostasis. Past the biochemical complexities, we'll likewise inspect what fasting means for irritation, oxidative pressure, and, surprisingly, the stomach microbiome—an expanding field of examination that reveals insight into the stomach-mind association and its effect on overall well-being. Through a mix of logical

examination and justifiable clarifications, this section equips you with a more profound perception of how fasting draws in our bodies on a subatomic level. As we explore the intricacies of healthful science, you'll acquire bits of knowledge that engage you to pursue informed decisions about when, why, and how to integrate fasting into your health process.

Chapter Three

The Psychological Odyssey: Fasting's Effect on Clearness and Concentration

In the advanced tornado of interruptions and requests, the journey for mental lucidity and an immovable centre has turned into a subtle pursuit. However, since the beginning of time, fasting has emerged as a strong impetus for honing the psyche and achieving uplifted mental states. This part takes us on a journey into the strange waters of fasting's significant effect on intelligence.

We navigate the scene of synapses and cerebrum capability, uncovering the perplexing manners by which fasting can invigorate the creation of neurotrophic factors that help mental strength. From the antiquated acts of yogic fasting to the cutting-edge peculiarity of irregular fasting, we examine the tales of people who have encountered improved fixation, imagination, and critical abilities to think through fasting.

Drawing on logical investigations and recounted proof, we investigate the possible connections between fasting and a further developed mindset, diminished pressure, and, surprisingly, a decreased risk of neurodegenerative problems. Through this psychological odyssey, we experience the peculiarity of "cerebrum haze" lifting, uncovering a more keen, more light-footed mind equipped for exploring the intricacies of the cutting-edge world.

As we dive further into the complexities of fasting's effect on intellectual capacities, we explore the domains of care and contemplation, uncovering the manners by which fasting can go about as an entry to elevated conditions of mindfulness and otherworldly understanding. Go along with us on this scholarly excursion as we disentangle the secrets of fasting's effect on the brain and find out how this antiquated practice can assist us with exploring the advanced mental scene with recharged clarity and concentration.

As of late, the interesting connection between fasting and mental clarity has earned consideration, igniting an enrapturing mental odyssey. Fasting, the act of avoiding nourishment for characterised periods, has been linked episodically to improved mental capability. As people set out on this excursion of self-disclosure, they dive into the possible effect of fasting on their clarity and concentration.

Although the logical investigation into the association between fasting and smartness is progressing, a few examinations have recommended that fasting could set off biochemical components like ketosis, which might improve mental execution. The idea of working on mental lucidity during fasting is charming, promising more keen concentration and increased mindfulness, much the same as a journey of the psyche towards freshly discovered clarity.

Be that as it may, this psychological odyssey isn't without its subtleties and intricacies. Individual encounters differ broadly, and factors like the span and kind of fasting, as well as a singular's special physiology, assume essential roles in forming the result. Talking with

Medical care experts must be consulted before setting out on this investigation to guarantee that the journey is left securely and capably.

As captivating as it could be, the psychological odyssey of fasting's effect on clarity and centre remaining parts is a domain where individual tales and arising logical bits of knowledge interlace. As explorers in this unfamiliar region, people proceed cautiously, looking for the expected mental advantages as well as a more profound comprehension of their personalities and bodies.

Note: This investigation fills in as an encouragement to think about the charming association between fasting and mental lucidity, underscoring the significance of both logical request and careful thought. As we explore this psychological odyssey, let us embrace the excursion with a receptive outlook and a promise of our prosperity.

Chapter Four

Otherworldly Aspects: Fasting as a Passage to Care

Past its physiological impacts, fasting has for quite some time been venerated as a sacrosanct practice that rises above the actual domain, filling in as a significant door to profound investigation and care. In this section, we set out on an excursion into the profound components of fasting, revealing how this well-established custom can extend our association with our internal identity and the more noteworthy universe.

We'll dive into the old insight of Eastern ways of thinking, where fasting has been used as a vehicle for achieving increased mindfulness and illumination. From the parsimonious acts of yogis to the thoughtful fasting customs of Buddhist priests, we'll investigate how fasting turns into a channel for developing presence, contemplation, and internal quietness.

Attracting equals to current pondering practices, we'll look at the job of fasting in working with care and opening further conditions of awareness. We'll explore the fragile interchange between fasting, contemplation, and care, uncovering how times of abstention can clear the psychological mess, permitting us to connect all the more completely with the current second.

All through this section, we'll experience accounts of otherworldly searchers who have tracked down comfort, disclosure, and a significant feeling of association through fasting. We'll ponder the force of purposeful hardship as a way to strip away interruptions and rediscover the quintessence of our reality.

Directed by insight into old practices and the experiences of contemporary otherworldliness, this part welcomes you to set out on a journey of self-revelation. As we cross the scene of fasting's otherworldly aspects,
you'll uncover the groundbreaking capability of this training in opening entryways to care, internal investigation, and a more profound fellowship with the secrets of life.
Past its physical and mental impacts, fasting has for some time been worshipped as a passage to significant otherworldly encounters and a method for extending one's association with one's internal identity and the
universe. This part leaves on a profound excursion, investigating how fasting turns into a vessel for care, contemplation, and otherworldly illumination.
We'll dig into the otherworldly customs where fasting assumes an urgent part, from the thoughtful acts of Buddhism to the pondering ceremonies of different beliefs. Through fasting, specialists look to rise above the constraints of the material world, opening themselves to uplifted conditions of mindfulness and otherworldly arousal.
The section likewise reveals how fasting can act as an impetus for ending up liberated from connections and propensities, cultivating a feeling of separation and freedom. As we investigate the tales of people who have embraced fasting ventures for the purpose of otherworldly investigation, we'll find the extraordinary force of quietness, isolation, and self-reflection.
Drawing upon the lessons of sages, spiritualists, and present-day profound pioneers, this part offers bits of knowledge about incorporating fasting as an instrument for care and inward development. Whether you're trying to develop your otherworldly practice or leave on a way of self-revelation, go along with us as we explore the domains of the spirit, uncovering how fasting turns into an entryway to the significant and profound elements of our reality.

Chapter Five

Fasting Methods: From Irregular Fasting to Expanded Restraint

As the old act of fasting finds its spot in the cutting-edge world, a different cluster of fasting methods arises, each offering a unique way to tackle its extraordinary potential. This section fills in as a thorough aid, unwinding the complexities of different fasting techniques that take special care of various ways of life, inclinations, and objectives.

We'll leave on an excursion through the domain of irregular fasting, investigating the well-known 16/8, 5:2, and eat-stop-eat approaches.

Disclosing the science behind these strategies, we'll comprehend what they mean for digestion, weight for executives, and, by and large, prosperity.

Wandering further, we'll dig into broadened fasting, where people avoid nourishment for longer periods, going from 24 hours to a few days.

From the actual difficulties to the psychological victories, we'll uncover the prizes and contemplations of leaving on these more serious fasting rehearsals.

Besides, we'll investigate changed fasting strategies, where the utilisation of explicit supplements or low-calorie food sources is permitted during fasting periods. These variations open roads for people who might have to explore fasting while at the same time overseeing ailments or explicit dietary prerequisites.

Whether you're attracted to the straightforwardness of irregular fasting or interested in the profundities of broadened restraint, this part furnishes you with the information and instruments to set out on your own fasting process. By understanding the complexities of every method, you'll be engaged to pick a fasting approach that lines up with your special requirements and yearnings, preparing for a way to well-being and imperativeness.

As the act of fasting keeps on enrapturing the cutting-edge world, a different cluster of fasting methods has arisen, each offering a remarkable way to deal with its advantages. In this section, we leave on an excursion through the range of fasting techniques, from the notable irregular fasting to the more broadened times of forbearance.

We'll disentangle the complexities of well-known fasting plans, like the 16/8 strategy, the 5:2 methodology, and the eat-stop-eat routine.

These procedures give an adaptable and versatile system for integrating fasting into different ways of life, empowering people to take advantage of the physical and mental advantages while obliging individual inclinations.

Digging further, we investigate the universe of broadened diets, where professionals stay away from nourishment for a few days or even weeks. From water diets to the delayed fasting-imitating diet, we'll reveal the possible advantages and contemplations related to longer fasting periods.

All through the section, we'll give useful directions on picking the fasting technique that lines up with your objectives, way of life, and well-being profile. We'll resolve normal inquiries, concerns, and misinterpretations, guaranteeing that you're outfitted with the information expected to set out on a fasting venture that impacts you.

Go along with us as we explore the ocean of fasting methods, uncovering the range of conceivable outcomes that engage you to make a fasting methodology customised to your exceptional desires and prosperity targets.

Chapter   Six
Powering Health: The Job of Nourishment in Fasting Cycles

In the unpredictable dance between fasting and devouring, sustenance assumes a vital role in expanding the advantages of the two states.

This part dives into the craft of sustenance during fasting cycles, investigating how careful food decisions can intensify the impacts of fasting and advance general prosperity.

We'll travel through the idea of supplement-rich eating,

uncovering the key supplements that help the body's versatility and imperativeness during fasting periods. From nutrients and minerals to cell reinforcements and fundamental unsaturated fats, we'll investigate how to make a decent and supportive eating routine that supplements your fasting routine.

Diving into the universe of pre-quick and post-quick feasts, we'll give commonsense bits of knowledge on setting up your body for fasting and changing out of it. Whether breaking a fast with painstakingly picked food

sources or supporting your body to support the advantages of fasting, we'll direct you through the sensitive course of powering well-being through insightful nourishment.

Drawing upon old insight and current nourishing science, this section offers a far-reaching manual for streamlining your eating examples to line up with your fasting cycles. By understanding the cooperative connection between fasting and sustenance, you'll be enabled to embark on an excursion of well-being that embraces the force of both forbearance and sustenance. Go along with us as we uncover the multifaceted woven artwork of nourishment inside the setting of fasting, enlightening the way to dynamic well-being and imperativeness.

While fasting is described by times of swearing off food, the transaction between sustenance and fasting cycles is critical for accomplishing ideal well-being and essentialness. This part plunges into the many-sided dance between nourishment and fasting, uncovering how what you eat during both fasting and taking care of periods can intensify the advantages of this training.

We'll investigate the idea of supplement thickness and its part in breaking a quick, featuring the significance of sustaining the body with healthy food varieties that give fundamental nutrients, minerals, and energy.

From breaking a quick with supplement-rich smoothies to adjusted feasts that support you through the fasting window, we'll offer functional experiences to fill your body shrewdly.

Moreover, we'll dig into the peculiarity of refeeding disorder, revealing insight into the potential dangers related to eating a lot of food excessively fast after a delayed fast. With a fair methodology, you can stay away from these traps and guarantee a consistent change among fasting and taking care of stages.

All through the part, we'll give recipes, feast-arranging tips, and dietary contemplations to assist you with upgrading the advantages of your fasting practice. By embracing the cooperative energy between nourishment and fasting, you'll be ready for upgraded prosperity and an amicable relationship with food.

Go along with us as we explore the scene of energising health, finding out how to figure out some kind of harmony among sustenance and fasting cycles to help your excursion towards well-being, imperativeness, and careful eating.

Chapter Seven

Defeating Difficulties: Methodologies for an Effective Fasting Experience

Leaving on a fasting excursion can be an extraordinary undertaking, yet it's not without its difficulties. In this part, we dive into the obstructions and barriers that might emerge during your fasting experience and give significant methodologies to assist you with exploring them with certainty and versatility.

We'll investigate the mental parts of fasting, including overseeing food cravings, adapting to desires, and developing a positive outlook. Through care strategies, mental reexamining, and functional tips, you'll acquire the instruments expected to defeat mental obstacles and remain enduring on your fasting path.

Furthermore, we'll address the social elements of fasting, offering direction on the most proficient method to convey your fasting objectives with friends and family, explore parties, and track down a steady local area to impart your excursion to. Fasting need not be a singular pursuit; by building an organisation of similar people, you can track down support and kinship en route.

Reasonable contemplations, for example, remaining hydrated, keeping up with electrolyte equilibrium, and checking your well-being all through the fasting system will likewise be investigated, guaranteeing your security and prosperity as you embrace this extraordinary practice.

With bits of knowledge from experienced specialists, master counsel, and an extensive tool compartment of techniques, this part prepares you to defeat difficulties, change misfortunes into valuable open doors, and accomplish an effective fasting experience that adds to your general prosperity.

Go along with us as we enlighten the way to win over

obstructions, engaging you to embrace the difficulties that accompany fasting and arise more grounded, smarter, and not set in stone to accomplish your well-being and essentialness objectives.

Leaving on a fasting excursion can be a groundbreaking

undertaking, yet it's not without its difficulties. In this section, we dig into the normal obstructions that people might experience during their fasting experience and give viable techniques to effectively explore them.

We'll address the physical and mental obstacles that might emerge, from overseeing cravings for food and desires to keeping up with inspiration and discipline. Through experiences established in social brain science and care procedures, we'll guide you in fostering a strong outlook that engages you to conquer hindrances and remain focused on your fasting objectives.

Additionally, we'll investigate how to fit fasting into various ways of life, tending to the necessities of competitors, shift labourers, and those with ailments. With customised approaches and viable counsel, you'll acquire the apparatus expected to adjust fasting to your remarkable conditions.

By digging into genuine accounts of people who have confronted and vanquished difficulties along their fasting process, this part plans to rouse and enable you to win over obstacles and embrace the groundbreaking capability of fasting. Go along with us as we outfit you with the systems and bits of knowledge to explore the exciting bends in the road of your fasting experience, changing difficulties into stepping stones toward a fruitful and improving fasting experience.

Chapter Eight

Fasting and Life Span: Investigating the Connections to a BetterLife

Chasing a more extended, better life, the act of fasting has emerged as a convincing road for upgrading life span and advancing in general prosperity. This part leaves off with an investigation of the intriguing association between fasting and life span, divulging the logical experiences and old insights that shed light on this extraordinary relationship.

We'll dive into the idea of caloric limitation and how it has been connected to broadening life expectancy in different creatures. By looking at the job of fasting in cell fix, DNA assurance, and mitochondrial capability, we'll uncover the systems through which fasting might contribute to deferring the maturing system.

Drawing upon the examination that has enlightened the impacts of fasting on markers of maturing, we'll investigate how discontinuous fasting and other fasting systems can possibly advance health span, permitting people to partake in an energetic and satisfying life as they age. We'll likewise dig into the idea of hormesis, where controlled stressors like fasting can enact versatile components that support flexibility and add to life span.

Directed by the insights of centenarians and current life span research, this section offers experiences into how fasting might be a vital aspect for opening the mysteries of a more drawn-out, really satisfying life.

Go along with us as we explore the intriguing landscape of fasting's effect on lifespan, divulging the pathways that might prompt an eventual fate of upgraded prosperity and essentialness.

In the journey for a more drawn-out, better life, fasting arises as an encouraging sign, promising to open the mysteries of broadened essentialness. This part leaves on an excursion into the interesting domain of fasting and life span, unwinding the logical proof and instruments behind the expected association.

We'll jump into the universe of caloric limitation, an idea that mirrors fasting's central rule, and look at its part in advancing life span by dialling back the maturing system and decreasing the risk of age-related illnesses. We'll investigate the impact of fasting on cell fix, irritation decrease, and the safeguarding of telomeres—basic markers of cell maturing.

Drawing on the discoveries of earth-shattering exploration and concentrating on creature models and people, we'll investigate the enticing possibilities of fasting as a methodology to expand health spans, the time of life set apart by essentialness and prosperity. We'll likewise address the debates and subtleties surrounding the point, giving a fair viewpoint on the possible advantages and constraints.

As we explore the scene of life span science, we'll engage you with experiences to help you pursue informed decisions about integrating fasting into your way of life with the end goal of living longer and, at the same time, living better. Go along with us as we venture through the complexities of fasting and its possible effect on the quest for a better, more energetic life.

Chapter Nine

Fasting Securely: Rules for Various Ways of Life and Ailments

While fasting holds various medical advantages, it's important to move toward this training with care and thought, particularly while managing different ways of life and ailments. In this part, we dive into the significance of fasting securely and give exhaustive rules customised to various conditions.

We'll investigate how factors, for example, age, orientation, movement level, and general well-being status, can impact your fasting process.

Whether you're a competitor looking for an execution upgrade or a person with explicit well-being concerns, we'll outfit you with bits of knowledge to settle on informed conclusions about the most reasonable fasting approach for your remarkable circumstance.

Moreover, we'll address the intersection of fasting and ailments, digging into the contemplations of people with diabetes, cardiovascular issues, hormonal irregularities, and other well-being challenges. With master counsel and proof-based suggestions, we mean to engage you to work with medical care experts to guarantee your fasting experience is both successful and safe.

Through genuine tributes and master experiences, this section gives a guide to exploring the intricacies of fasting while at the same time accommodating different ways of life and well-being needs. Go along with us as we venture toward a comprehensive comprehension of fasting security, encouraging a mindful and very educated way to deal with the advantages of this groundbreaking practice.

Guaranteeing a protected fasting experience is paramount, particularly as fasting acquires prevalence among people with different ways of life and clinical foundations. In this part, we dig into the urgent subject of fasting security, offering common sense rules and bits of knowledge to explore fasting ventures customised to explicit conditions.

We'll investigate contemplations for various age groups, from youngsters to more seasoned adults, featuring what fasting might mean for development, advancement, and age-related well-being concerns. Also, we'll address the requirements of pregnant and breastfeeding people, revealing insight into the fragile harmony between fasting and maternal and foetal prosperity.

Understanding that ailments differ broadly, we'll give bits of knowledge on how fasting can be adjusted for people with diabetes, cardiovascular issues, and other well-being challenges. We'll likewise address the expected collaborations among fasting and drugs, underscoring the significance of counselling medical care experts before rolling out critical improvements to one's fasting schedule.

All through the section, our point is to engage you with the information expected to help you come to informed conclusions about fasting in a manner that focuses on your well-being and prosperity. By exploring the perplexing landscape of fasting security, you'll be prepared to set out on a fasting venture that lines up with your remarkable conditions and needs.

Go along with us as we unwind the embroidered artwork of fasting security, offering direction that engages you to move toward fasting with certainty and care, guaranteeing that your process isn't just groundbreaking but additionally protected and enhanced.

Chapter Ten

Tributes: Genuine Accounts of Change and Mending

In the embroidered artwork of human encounters, fasting has woven strings of significant change and recuperation. In this section, we uncover the voices of people whose lives have been moved by fasting, sharing their real and motivating accounts of progress, development, and victory.

Through these individual tributes, we'll travel close to people who have outfit fasting to beat difficulties, from weight battles for executives to constant medical issues. These accounts give testimony regarding the force of fasting to lighten versatility, open internal strength, and cultivate a reestablished sense of direction.

By sharing firsthand records, we mean to overcome any issues among hypotheses and work on them, offering a brief look into the present reality of the effect of fasting on different lives. These stories exhibit the potential for actual restoration, mental lucidity, and profound improvement that lie on the opposite side of a fasting venture.

As we dive into the lived encounters of these people, we welcome you to draw motivation and understanding from their ways of changing. Whether you're leaving on your own fasting journey or looking for approval and consolation, these tributes act as a demonstration of the limitless capability of fasting to cultivate significant recuperating and enduring change.

Behind each training lies an embroidery of individual stories, each winding around a one-of-a-kind story of change and recuperation. In this part, we turn the focus on people who have set out on their own fasting processes, sharing their genuine tributes of how fasting has impacted their lives in significant ways.

From weight reduction and working on metabolic well-being to mental lucidity and profound arousal, these accounts act as reference points of motivation, representing the different ways in which fasting can shape our prosperity. Through the expressions of the individuals who have gone through the fasting experience, we gain bits of knowledge about the difficulties they've survived, the illustrations they've learned, and the advantages they've procured.

By exhibiting a scope of points of view and results, this part highlights the fact that there is no one-size-fits-all way to deal with fasting. All things being equal, every individual's process is an exceptional investigation that unfolds against the backdrop of their own conditions, wants, and goals.

Go along with us as we drench ourselves in the embroidered artwork of human experience, finding the groundbreaking force of fasting through the eyes of the people who have left on this excursion of self-disclosure, restoration, and mending.

The excursion of fasting is set apart by private stories that enlighten the force of this training to change lives, lighten mending, and motivate significant change. In this part, we present an assortment of genuine tributes from people who have set out on their own fasting processes, sharing their surprising accounts of victory over difficulties and the revelation of freshly discovered prosperity.

From weight reduction wins to mental clarity leaps, every tribute gives a brief look into the different ways in which fasting has impacted the lives of individuals from varying backgrounds. Through their words, you'll observe firsthand the effect of fasting on actual well-being, mental versatility, and profound equilibrium.

These accounts act as a wellspring of motivation and strengthening, offering an engaging and legitimate point of view on the delights and battles that go with the way to well-being and essentialness through fasting. As you

read about the groundbreaking encounters of others, you'll track down reverberation, support, and a feeling of the local community that builds up the capability of fasting to achieve good change.

Go along with us as we plunge into the genuine accounts of people who have tackled the force of fasting to change their accounts, demonstrating that this antiquated practice keeps on holding the way to opening the potential for change and mending in our advanced lives.

Chapter Eleven

Beyond the Fast: Incorporating Fasting into Day-to-Day Existence

As the limits between fasting and day-to-day existence obscure, another section of investigation unfurls—one where fasting turns out to be something other than a training, but a lifestyle. In this section, we dive into the craft of coordinating fasting into the texture of regular presence, manufacturing an amicable connection between sustenance, prosperity, and the rhythms of present-day living.

We'll investigate the idea of careful eating, directing you to the most proficient method to relish and value every piece, whether during fasting or taking care of periods. We'll reveal the job of fasting in reshaping your relationship with food, encouraging a more profound comprehension of yearning signs, close-to-home eating, and satiety.

Also, we'll inspect how fasting can impact social elements and connections, offering techniques to convey your fasting process to companions, family, and partners while encouraging an air of help and regard.

From common sense tips for dinner arranging and using time productively to methods for keeping up with fasting during movement and exceptional events, this section furnishes you with the apparatuses to flawlessly mesh fasting into the woven artwork of your day-to-day routine. By embracing fasting not as a different undertaking but rather as an indispensable piece of your comprehensive prosperity, you'll leave on an extraordinary excursion that reaches beyond simple abstention, prompting a reasonable, deliberate, and improved approach to everyday life.

Go along with us as we step into the domain of coordinated fasting, investigating the vast capability of fitting this training with the musicality of ordinary presence.

As the pages of this book unfold, you've ventured through the set of experiences, science, and extraordinary capabilities of fasting. Presently, we turn our concentration to the craft of coordinating fasting into your day-to-day presence, guaranteeing that its advantages reach a long way beyond the bounds of a particular fasting window.

In this section, we investigate how fasting can become a vital part of your way of life, consistently meshing into your schedules, propensities, and decisions. We'll dig into systems for keeping up with the advantages of fasting in any event during times of eating, stressing the significance of careful sustenance and adjusted eating designs.

We'll likewise address the idea of recurrent fasting, where irregular fasting is woven into the ordinary musicality of life, adjusting to the back-and-forth movement of your day-to-day requests. Whether you're

exploring parties, work responsibilities, or travel, we'll give you insights into how to explore these situations while remaining consistent with your fasting objectives.

Besides, we'll investigate the cooperative connection between fasting and all-encompassing prosperity, including rest, cleanliness, stress for executives, and exercise. By encouraging a coordinated way to deal with

well-being, you'll find that fasting fills in as a foundation for general imperativeness and an agreeable way of life.

As you embrace the insight of this section, you'll uncover the way to flawlessly integrate the standards of fasting into the embroidered artwork of your daily existence. Go along with us as we set out on an excursion that rises above fasting's limits, engaging you to saddle its advantages as you explore the intricacies of current living.

Chapter Twelve

Recipes for Restoration: Nutrient-Rich Meals to Break the Fast

Breaking a fast is a snapshot of expectation and opportunity, a chance to feed the body with healthy, supplement-rich food varieties that help its revival and renewal. In this section, we present a variety of delightful recipes carefully organised to give you a sustaining and fulfilling experience as you break your quick.

From energetic and supplement-stuffed smoothie bowls overflowing with cell reinforcements to protein-rich servings of mixed greens enhanced with bright vegetables, every recipe is intended to consistently progress your body from a fasting state to one of sustenance. We'll investigate the ideal equilibrium of macronutrients and micronutrients to guarantee ideal processing and energy.

For those investigating different dietary inclinations, we've made recipes that take care of the scope of requirements, including veggie lovers, vegetarians, and omnivores. Whether you're looking for a good breakfast

or a light noontime feast to break your fast, these recipes offer a range of flavours and textures to please your sense of taste.

With bit-by-bit guidelines, cooking tips, and an understanding of the dietary benefit of each dish, this part engages you to settle on educated and heavenly decisions while breaking your quick. Go along with us as we set out on a culinary excursion that entices your taste buds as well as enhances your prosperity, making each feast a festival of restoration and imperativeness.

Breaking a quick isn't just about fulfilling hunger; it's a

valuable chance to feed your body with thick food varieties that renew and rejuvenate. In this section, we dig into the domain of culinary imagination,

offering an organised assortment of recipes intended to upgrade your fasting experience and advance a lively feeling of prosperity.

From stimulating smoothie bowls to good plates of mixed greens overflowing with variety and flavour, our recipes are painstakingly created to give an amicable mix of fundamental supplements while taking special care of different dietary inclinations. Each dish is nicely adjusted to help assimilation, advance energy levels, and light your taste buds with enchantment.

Whether you're breaking a short discontinuous fast or a more broadened time of restraint, these recipes act as a culinary ally to your fasting process. We'll give bit-by-bit guidelines, fixes for replacements, and customization tips, enabling you to make sustaining feasts that line up with your inclinations and requirements.

As you investigate the flavours and surfaces of these supplement-rich recipes, you'll find that breaking a fast can be a chance for both actual restoration and gastronomic delight. Go along with us on a culinary experience that commends the speciality of sustenance and adds a dynamic new aspect to your fasting experience.

Breaking a fast is a valuable chance to support your body with healthy and thick food sources that complement the advantages of fasting. In this section, we investigate an organised assortment of reviving recipes intended to empower your faculties, support your prosperity, and praise the craft of careful eating.

From energetic and bright smoothie bowls overflowing with cell reinforcements to good and fulfilling servings of mixed greens overflowing with protein and fibre, our recipes offer a range of choices to suit different preferences and inclinations. We'll direct you through the planning of adjusted dinners that give fundamental supplements, assisting you with progressing from fasting to taking care of your beauty and goals.

Every recipe is thoughtfully made to give sustenance, energy, and a brilliant culinary encounter. Whether you're looking for post-quick hydration, maintainable fuel, or a culinary experience that entices your taste buds, our assortment of recipes will motivate you to commend the breaking of your quick in a way that upholds your general prosperity.

Go along with us as we set out on a culinary investigation, revealing the speciality of making supplement-rich feasts that amicably line up with your fasting process, guaranteeing that your sustenance after a quick is as reviving and fulfilling as the fasting experience itself.

Chapter Thirteen

Embracing a Fresh Start: Your Customised Fasting Excursion

As you've explored through the sections of this book, you've acquired experiences in the diverse universe of fasting—it's set of experiences, science, otherworldly aspects, and functional applications.

Presently, furnished with information and motivation, now is the ideal time to embark on your own one-of-a-kind fasting venture, one that is customised to your objectives, inclinations, and yearnings.

In this finishing-up part, we guide you through the most common way of making a fasting plan that resounds with your singular requirements.

We'll give you apparatus for setting clear aims, making reasonable objectives, and keeping tabs on your development. Whether you're looking to work on actual

well-being, mental lucidity, or otherworldly development, this section offers a guide to assist you with saddling the maximum capacity of fasting in a presence that array with your perception.

Through self-reflection, directed prompts, and master

exhortation, you'll be engaged to plan a maintainable fasting schedule that coordinates flawlessly with your way of life. We'll urge you to move toward

your fasting process with an open heart and a feeling of interest, embracing the potential chance to learn, adjust, and develop as you explore the way to well-being and essentialness.

Go along with us as we commend the unfolding of a fresh start—your customised fasting venture—and set out on an extraordinary experience that holds the commitment of development, prosperity, and an extra intelligent alliance with yourself and your broad enclosing.

As you venture through the pages of this book, you've acquired experiences into the set of experiences, science, and extraordinary capability of fasting. Presently, the opportunity has arrived to set out on your own customised fasting venture—a journey that holds the commitment of prosperity, essentialness, and self-disclosure.

In this section, we guide you through the most common way of making a fasting plan custom-made to your unique goals, way of life, and well-being profile. We'll assist you with putting forth reasonable objectives, selecting the fasting techniques that impact you, and coordinating fasting consistently into your schedules.

Through self-evaluation activities and reflection prompts, you'll acquire clarity on your inspirations, challenges, and desired results.

Outfitted with this mindfulness, you'll be better prepared to explore your fasting process with reason and aim, embracing every second as a chance for development and change.

We'll address the significance of self-sympathy and adaptability, advising you that your process is remarkably yours and that progress is set apart by your victories and misfortunes. With masterful direction and reasonable guidance, you'll feel engaged to assume responsibility for your well-being, imperativeness, and prosperity as you step into this fresh start.

Go along with us as we guide you through the most common way of making a customised fasting venture that lines up with your vision of a better, more dynamic life. With each step you take, you'll embrace another section as well as a significant chance for self-revelation and enduring change.

Conclusion :

Embracing the Embroidery of Fasting's True Capacity

As we arrive at the last pages of "Fasting: The Path To Health and Vitality," we end up at the junction of antiquated intelligence and present-day disclosure. The excursion through fasting has been one of investigation, edification, and change—a journey that has risen above reality to enlighten the multitude of ways in which fasting can enhance our lives.

From the authentic foundations of fasting across societies and periods to its significant effect on actual well-being, mental lucidity, and profound development, we've dug into the profundities of this training. We've
investigated the science behind its consequences for the body, the brain, and the spirit, uncovering the multifaceted components that underlie its power.

We've explored the difficulties and wins of fasting, furnishing you with procedures to beat impediments and embrace the potential for mending and prosperity. We've commended the tales of genuine people whose lives have been everlastingly changed by their fasting processes, offering a demonstration of the flexibility of the human soul.

As you stand at the limit of your own customised fasting

venture, recall that the way you tread is one of probability, development, and self-disclosure. With the information you've acquired and the direction you've taken, you hold the key to opening the groundbreaking capability of fasting—training that can reshape your well-being, your mentality, and your association with your general surroundings.

May this book act as a wellspring of motivation, strengthening, and support as you leave on your own extraordinary journey to well-being and imperativeness through fasting. Embrace the embroidery of fasting's true capacity, and may your process be loaded up with recharging, strength, and a reestablished vitality.

Goodbye, dear peruser, and may your fasting process be as enhancing and extraordinary as the tales that have unfurled inside these pages.